STONE PEOPLE MEDICINE

by

Manny Twofeathers

X

Wo-Pila Publishing
Phoenix, Arizona

Printed and bound in the U.S.A.

First printing 1997

Although the author has tried to ensure the accuracy and
completeness of the information contained in this book, we
assume no responsibility for errors, inaccuracies, omissions
or any inconsistency herein. Any slights of people or
organizations are unintentional.

Twofeathers, Manny
          Stone People Medicine

ISBN 1-886340-97-8

TABLE OF CONTENTS

Page

SECTION II SPIRIT ANIMAL/ FIGURES 55

ACKNOWLEDGEMENTS

First I want to thank the Spirits for the guidance they brought me. The stones have given me all I need to make this book interesting and informational. I honor both entities.

May the Spirits always bless my wife, Melody for all the hours spent on the computer. Sitting there without a word, changing and adjusting the book until I was happy. Without you this book wouldn't have happened.

My deepest thanks to my dear friend and sis, Marlene O'Connor for all the times she's helped us and put up with my demands. Also Carla Treatch and Cary Mungai for all their help keeping me straight and not letting our business go down the tubes. Thanks much!

Last but not least I want to thank my girls for putting up with me while I was writing. I was pretty impossible at times. Thanks Stormy, Mary, Becky, Dory and Oriona.

And to my new son, "Stone," who couldn't be born until this book was done!

STONE PEOPLE
MEDICINE

The contents of this book are solely my beliefs. I am not implying this is the belief of any Native American tribe or any group of people. What I talk about in this book are things I have learned by experience, from the elders I've talked to and from the Spirits that brought me help and wisdom when I needed it. The stones work for me and what I've gained in knowledge and spirituality from them I'm willing to share with you. I believe my spiritual awakening and knowledge is a direct result of my learning to listen and communicate with both the stones and the spirits. I'm not suggesting what has happened to me, will also happen to everyone that reads this book. My sincere wishes are whoever reads this book will benefit from my experiences. They can learn how to use the stones and animal spirits to help themselves spiritually, emotionally and even financially. It's my intention to show you how to find a better way of life.

INTRODUCTION

1. How Stone People came into
   my life

It seems the Stone People have been with me all my life. I remember when I was very young, picking up stones and coming home with pockets full of them. On wash day, my mom would take my pants outside and shake them, holding them upside down. There was always a small pile of stones right next to the back door of our old house. Growing up in Ajo, Arizona, a copper mining town, kept my interest in stones and rocks alive for all of my youth and continues still today.

While working on this book, my family and I were in Ajo visiting my mom, sisters and brother. Telling them about stones and how important they are, I mentioned this book. I said I couldn't understand why I had always been interested in stones. Without saying a word my mom walked into her bedroom. Returning she handed me a small stone. She explained that it had belonged to her mother. My grandmother passed away when my mom was four years of age. That was the only thing my mom had left from her mother. We don't know how long she had the stone. We estimate it has been in the family at least eighty years. A lot of people would not consider it a beautiful stone. However it has one distinct characteristic, no matter how hot the temperature is, it always remains cool. Beautiful or not, to me it means more than any other stone that's ever come to me. It tells me where my interest in stones comes from. I sit and hold it, hoping it will bring me something from my grandmother. If nothing else it brings me comfort.

In later years I had painted native figures on small flat rocks, and sold a few. Unfortunately, it wasn't as popular as I had hoped. I slowly sold the stones I had painted and my interest moved to other things. At the time I felt sad because I had been working with small flat rocks that felt good to me. They had a way of calming me down. Sadly, because they weren't profitable, I let them drift out of my life. In retrospect I feel if I would have stayed with them, they would have rewarded me by becoming good sellers. I was just too impatient to wait.

Through the years stones have been

coming in to and going out of my life. However the first time that stones had a very profound impact on me was in a Sweat Lodge Ceremony shortly before my first Sundance in Fort Washakie, Wyoming. Sweat Lodges are small, low, hut-like structures made of willow branches. It's covered with whatever materials are available such as canvas, blankets etc. Rocks heated hot enough to turn them red in a fire pit are put into the Sweat Lodge. Water is poured on the hot rocks, after they're brought in, to create steam. This serves as purification for those in the Sweat Lodge.

This was something new and strange to me. As I followed a friend of mine on our hands and knees into it, a pleasant sense of peace, embraced me inside the Sweat Lodge. It felt as though I had reached a summit in my life. When we stopped crawling, I took my place in the Sweat Lodge in what was to be my new space in a new life. After a few minutes of silence my friend started talking slowly. He explained things to me about the Sweat Lodge, why we were doing it, what it did for us. He explained many things I knew nothing about. I listened to all he was saying, and didn't want to miss anything. Knowing deep inside that what I was learning was forever and what was coming to me would change my life, in a very big way.

Finally he asked the fire keeper to bring in the first stone. It created a very special moment for me. As each large stone was brought in and placed in the pit, the heat increased, inside the Sweat Lodge. It was a comforting feeling, as though I was stepping into my mother's home once again. I saw faces in each of the Grandfather rocks, as though they were smiling and welcoming me home. As I sat there with the others, the heat from the rocks and the quietness inside the lodge was relaxing. It was quiet and comforting inside.

From outside I could hear a bird happily chirping. It felt as though I had crawled into another world, another dimension. One of complete safety. Yet hearing the bird outside allowed me the perspective of knowing that I was still in the material world. So I waited. Holding my breath for whatever was to come next. What I received that day in the Sweat Lodge was a deep satisfied feeling of contentment. The stones had given me a clearly defined direction to my life. Slowly I started to understand the message coming to me from the stones.

Then one day in 1992, while on a sales call in Toronto, the Stone People tried to get my attention. My wife Melody and I walked into one of our customer's stores. During the course of our conversation, the manager of the store and good friend, asked me if I had ever thought of painting animals on rocks. Smiling, I told him I had in the past, on small flat rocks. He pulled a small round stone out of his pocket and showed me what he meant.

I looked at it but didn't see it, passing it off as insignificant or too hard to do. My memory of what my thoughts were at the moment is unclear. Something had clicked but I ignored it.

Several days passed then I guess the spirits decided to give me another chance at finding out what they were trying to show me.

That night I dreamed that I was visited by four different animals. After seeing each one I would see the Grandfather rocks in the Sweat Lodge. First I saw an Eagle. Then I saw not one, but many Buffalo running. The next ones to come to me were the Spider and the Otter. Several days after the first dream four other animals came to me. A Snake and a Bear appeared, then a Turtle and a Wolf. Each time I would see the Grandfather rocks in the Sweat Lodge. Seeing the animals then the rocks in the Sweat Lodge started taking a familiar pattern.

Often, while making our crafts with

my family, I would think of all eight animals. My thoughts would drift as I sat there. I would see these animals that had come to me in dreams. It was becoming second nature to see the animals and relate them to stones. But I still didn't see the connection of putting animal pictures on stones.

Suddenly, I would remember the encounter at the store with my friend. Then remembering, my dreams would take over my thoughts. It seemed that all it took was one thought that triggered another and another until it came full circle to the stones and the animals. The spirits kept trying to bring the animals and stones to my attention. I guess they already knew how well they would help a lot of people. I'm glad the spirits were persistent. They really must have thought I was dense for not getting it.

Thoughts of stones and animals would weave their way in and out of my mind. What I was being told was how each animal was to help people. The animal's pictures should be on the stones. With the combined strength of the animal spirits and the wisdom of the stones, this knowledge would belong to whoever had the stone. This was the only way both could be together at once. I started writing down what I was told, while listening to my thoughts. Finally I knew I had all the information I needed to start doing the Stone People Medicine stones. I was even brought the name for them. The eight animals are the ones we put on stones.

The other two did not come to me in dreams but I feel they had to be done because of the help they can give others. Being from the southwest I had always been familiar with Kokopelli and the Man-in-the-Maze. So we added them to our list.

Soon after the dreams and making the connection to the stones, I got some paints and small round stones and started painting the animals on the stones. Stone People Medicine was officially born.

My family and I spent hours looking for small stones on the shores of Lake Ontario, Canada. In the beginning I was hand drawing on each stone, one at a time. It was a slow and tedious chore. The demand for my little stones started growing. I'm very grateful that people thought enough of them to keep buying them while I learned and got used to doing them. I had to start producing them faster and faster, but I never forgot to pray and to be thankful for the good things coming to us because of them.

The small stones that we now use as our Stone People Medicine come from the western ocean beaches. They are volcanic, and were blown into the ocean thousands of years ago. The constant wave movement has gently tumbled and smoothed the sharp edges of each stone. This gives them all a smooth, soft touch. The energy from the volcano (fire), combined with the ocean (water) waves, gives the stones a nice balance of energy.

Then tragedy struck. My eyesight started to deteriorate. Native Americans are very susceptible to diabetes, and I am no exception. I don't know if that's the reason for the problem with my eyes but I know that I do have a problem. It devastated me. Once again I had to go to the stones and spirits with my prayers, for guidance. There had to be a way to duplicate my art work so that my children could help me.

So I prayed and the stones and spirits showed me the way. They guided me to the right people that could help me. They showed me that I didn't have to actually paint each and every stone. As long as each stone was hand picked, in a good way.

I ask everyone who helps with the making of these stones to always try to be in a good and cheerful mood. To not be angry or upset when working with the Stone People Medicine. I ask if they don't feel good, to stay away from them until they feel better.

There is a good reason I do this. Just as one person can affect others, they can affect the stones. I believe stones are also living entities, it might affect the way the little stones help others if contaminated by bad energy. Within the shape of each stone the molecules are constantly moving as they do in our bodies. That is the reason I believe that they are also as alive as we are.

2. Why they are significant today.

Stones have been helping people through the ages, and they continue to do so today. You as the person receiving the help, and knowledge must make an effort to receive by being open and believing that they will help you. This, as simple as it may sound, is why they play such a significant role in our lives.

Perhaps the reason people need this type of spiritual object is due to the fact that many today are spiritually bankrupt. Some of the established religions aren't giving people what they need. Many people today need hope, and some feel they have nothing tangible to hold on to.

These stones we are talking about, are not the ones mentioned throughout the Bible. We believe that they have as much to offer as any stone in the universe, if it comes to you. Stone Peopie Medicine can be a solid object to hold on to and send one's prayers, dreams, hopes and wishes to the creator.

From Ajo, as a child to the Sweat Lodge Ceremony in Wyoming and to this day, Stone People have been a big influence on me all my life. During the Sweat Lodge they had a very profound impact on me, both physically and spiritually. I feel that they were the solid bridge that helped me span the gap between the physical and spiritual worlds.

SECTION I
STONE PEOPLE

Why did the Old People think that stones were so important?

Why do so many believe that they are sacred?

Why are all people, adults and even children so attracted to stones?

Why have we used stones for ceremonies for so many centuries?

Why do we place such high value on some of them and not others?

Why do some people believe in stones so much, that they use them for divining the future, or as special talismans - even for healing?

Every month has a birthstone. Where does the belief come from?

Through the ages people of knowledge have used stones for

inspiration and guidance.

I could go on and on with these kinds of questions, but I ask all this because I want you to stop and think about stones and what you're about to learn. It is my belief that the stones themselves bring us the knowledge on how to use them to our benefit.

Not only native people from here honor and respect stones. People from all over the world have done so for thousands of years.

Because Stone People are not moving, does that mean they have no life? Isn't it true the molecules in stones are always moving just as they are moving in our human bodies? Stones, I believe are another form of life, just like all plants, water and even the wind. I believe they are all different forms of life. But right now our only interest is in stones.

In comparison to the lives of the Stone People, our lives are like shooting stars racing a turtle. It is my belief that Stone People are not even aware we exist. To them we move so fast, we must only be a shrill, buzzing irritation. The slowness of the Stone Peoples lives, gives them the time and ability to gather knowledge and wisdom. That's where we come in, we have got to slow ourselves down and reap what they have to offer.

Stones or rocks are the original material of our Mother Earth. Without it nothing else could have followed in creation. Our stones here on earth are a piece of a much larger picture. The earth is also a little piece of the universe. It stands to reason, the stones that make our earth, also carry within them the knowledge of the universe. That knowledge is there for the taking. It's there for those, willing to learn, to listen and put the knowledge into practice. This can be your personal crash course on how to gain everything you ever wanted.

1. Stones most used by native people.

There are three main stones that were extremely important to native people. They are Pipestone for the Sacred Pipe, Obsidian and Flint for making arrowheads and tools.

Pipestone was first quarried around sixteen hundred by the Iowa and Oto tribes. In later years the sites where it is quarried came into the possession of the Lakota people. To this day most of the people that work the quarries are Lakota. There are people of different tribes also willing to go through the very difficult work of extracting this beautiful stone.

It is mainly used for making ceremonial pipe bowls. The pipe is used in spiritual ceremonies. It is believed that the pipe smoke carries prayers and messages to the Great Spirit.

Though ceremonial pipe bowls are the main objects carved from it, there are many native artists who use Pipestone to create other objects of art. They carve small bears, turtles, and other beautiful pieces. The reason this came about is that there was a lot of Pipestone that was too thin to make bowls out of and we hated to see it going to waste. So many other things are made from it today. The quarrying of Pipestone in Minnesota is reserved only for Native Americans of all tribes. I personally had my own quarry at one time, but because of my age and the difficulty of getting the stone out, I let my permit expire.

Obsidian is recognized by native

people as the symbol of a Warrior. It can be chipped down to the width of a molecule. It is volcanic glass and was used for making tools, arrowheads and knives for cutting meat and skinning game. Recently, an arrowhead was found, and was estimated to be around 2.5 million years old. It's good to know my ancestors have been here in this hemisphere so many years and have been connected with stones for such a long time. Psychic Surgeons from the Philippines and healers from Central and South America were known to use Obsidian tools in surgery.

There is also a mention in the bible, (Exodus chapter 4, verse 25) when a sharp stone was used for circumcision. Could it have been Obsidian or Flint stone they used? Flint can be chipped to the same sharpness as Obsidian. To my knowledge there are no other stones on earth that can be chipped to this degree. Flint stone was found mostly in the eastern part of the country. Obsidian was found mostly in the west.

Today both kinds of arrowheads and artifacts are found all over the country. The old people loved to trade not only hides, food, sea shells, but also weapons. Arrows and war clubs made from both materials were traded or changed ownership during battles between different tribes. I have personally found a beautiful war club head in Arizona. An anthropologist told me the stone it was made from, can only be found east of the Mississippi river. I always wondered how it got to where I found it, in the middle of Arizona!

There are some Aztec traditions that say if you put a piece of Obsidian in a container of water, then after twenty-four hours remove the stone. Drink the water. It will purify, heal and protect you.

It isn't just the stones I have mentioned that are useful to us. The old native medicine people would use many different kinds of stones. They were used in interpreting life or seeking direction for others.

For us today, a stone coming into your life, I believe has something significant or some knowledge for you. You must listen. That stone can be bought, found or it might come to you as a gift. When the feeling comes to you, it is also a very wonderful feeling to give one as a gift. If inspired to give one, remember the stone has something to give the person its going to. The stone is using you as transportation to that person.

2. Spiritual beliefs and uses

There are many references in different religious texts that refer to stones. Some biblical examples are in the book of Exodus, chapter 28, verses 17-22. God tells Moses to create a breastplate for his brother Aaron. The breastplate was to contain twelve stones, here are a few of them: topaz, emerald, sapphire, diamond, agate, amethyst, onyx and jasper. The twelve stones were supposed to represent the twelve tribes of Israel.

Moses "went up on the hill" on Mount Sinai to receive guidance. Was he in fact going on a "vision quest" as native people do? He was receiving guidance from God. Was he possibly receiving guidance from the Stone People also? He was given the laws from God or ten commandments on stone tablets (Exodus, Chapter 20).

The stone tablets were said to be made of lapis lazuli. This has become known as the Stone of the Heavens, because God used it to write his laws. The deep blue color represents the heavens and the golden flecks of pyrite, the stars.

In Revelations, Chapter 21, the twelve foundations of the New Jerusalem, each foundation was a precious stone, jasper, sapphire, chalcedony, emerald, sardonyx, sardius, chrysolite, beryl, topaz, chrysoprase, jacinth and amethyst. Why are these particular stones significant? Did they possess supernatural properties, or other powers? Or did they contain wisdom and knowledge for those that were around them and were ready to receive that knowledge? Did the old Spiritual leaders know of the powers of the stones? Was this knowledge kept for the exclusive use of only a few? Were the stones in fact the place where they drew their wisdom from?

Ah!! So many questions and so few answers.

In my book, "The Road to the Sundance," I explain how my second Sundance in Wyoming in 1986, brought me a vision. My vision told me how I was going to be able to help people in all directions some day. I was told that a medicine man would bring me the information when the time was right.

In the summer of 1992, after I finished Sundancing for the day, a medicine man came to my camp to talk. He had a message for me from the spirits. Two stones would be coming to me he said and I was to use them for healing. He explained that they wouldn't be crystals, just common stones, but I would know when they came to me. When the time was right, the spirits would bring me the knowledge on how to use them.

I thought it was strange he was telling me that because ironically, we made part of our living from small stones called, "Stone People Medicine."

Now it's several years later, a very profound realization has come to me. When the spirits told me I would be helping people in all the directions, I thought it was to be "one on one" type of help. It was hard to see how I could physically help so many. The realization is that, I personally will not help all these people, but what I write and how I write my books will be what helps people in all directions. When that knowledge came to me, a great deal of pressure was lifted from my soul. I have become more determined in my quest for spiritual knowledge, and for the correctness of everything I write.

Two weeks later, while in Memphis, Tennessee I called an old friend of mine and his wife. They invited us to their home and prepared a breakfast feast for my family. After breakfast, he took me aside and told me he had something for me. He gave me a stone, and explained that he was a stone man. This means he is responsible for giving people stones when they need them. People like him are picked by the Spirits to help others. They are picked through dreams and visions they have. I hadn't said anything about what had happened at the Sundance. He didn't know anything about the other Sundancer that had brought me the message. Now here he was giving me my first stone.

A week later, while at a pow wow in Columbus, Ohio, we were set up selling our crafts. A woman who was set up next to us came to me with tears in her eyes. She handed me this unusual stone. She said a month before she was at a Sundance in Ontario, Canada supporting her son. Something told her to pick up this stone. She somehow knew it was for someone else. She explained that she didn't like the stone and thought it was ugly, but was still told to keep it and she listened. Seeing me, she knew I was the person it was meant for. At the time she was emotional, realizing the spirits had used her for something very special. Again it came to me, just as I was told. Not long after that, I was to put these stones to use.

After that pow wow, we left for Maryland and attended another small Sundance. Though a day late, I went in the Sundance to help. I was told one of the dancers, had been laying on the ground since the Sundance had started two days before with a powerful migraine headache. He was completely incapacitated by the pain, and was violently ill the entire time he was under the arbor.

Though reluctant at first, I felt that the spirits had put me in this situation so I would use the stones to help him.

Getting the dancer to get up was almost impossible, due to the pain. Three other Sundancers were there to help me with him. His mouth was salivating from the pain. He was carried into the Sweat Lodge for healing. At first I didn't know what to do, so I sat there and waited for the spirits to guide me. What happened in there is not to be repeated outside the Sweat Lodge. The spirits guided me through my thoughts on what to do. When it was over, I was shown how powerful this medicine is. Within half an hour the Sundancer that received the healing, came to me with a gift, a smile and clear eyes. He thanked me and said, "I don't know what medicine you use, but keep using it, you'll help others. My headache is completely gone." Would his headache have left him if I hadn't done what I did?

Though many believe if you talk about the medicine brought to you, you will lose it. When you share and show people your medicine, I believe you are helping others to help themselves. Using the medicine to help others, is the reason it was brought to you. This brings forth an important quote by **Nelson** Mandela, as follows:

*"Our deepest fear is not that we are inadequate. Our deepest fear is that we are powerful beyond measure. It is our light, not our darkness, that frightens us. We ask ourselves, who am I to be brilliant, gorgeous, talented and fabulous? Actually, who are you **not** to be? You are a child of God. Your playing small doesn't serve the world. There's nothing enlightened about shrinking so that other people won't*

feel insecure around you. We were born to manifest the glory of God within us. It's not just some of us, it's in everyone. And as we let our light shine, we unconsciously give other people permission to do the same. As we are liberated from our own fear, our presence automatically liberates others."

When I read this piece of wisdom, it seemed to lighten the load on my mind and spirit, and brought much joy into my life. I knew it also affected others around me, and affected what I had to write. It is exactly what I have always wanted to say. I just didn't have the inspiration that prompted Mr. Mandela. What he says is very timely for my book, "The Road to the Sundance" because I was told by the Spirits that I had to share the experiences and visions of my life with everyone. It's also very timely for this book. This book will teach you how to come out of your shell and not be afraid to help yourself and to help others. Finally, I had realized my vision from so long ago. I guess the spirits felt I was ready. They had shown me the power of the stones, and how this medicine would be my way to help others.

Returning to Toronto after the Sundance, that fall I woke up one morning with a sharp pain in my upper abdomen. For the next four days the pain kept getting worse and worse. Writing it off as indigestion, or heartburn, eventually I realized it must be something more serious. Melody, my wife kept trying to get me to go to the hospital. I kept refusing, until the pain became unbearable. Agreeing to go to the hospital, I asked Melody to give me a few minutes alone.

I was going to attempt to use the stones on myself. Though fearful of failing, I had to see if it would work on me. I laid down and waited for the spirits to guide me. After a few moments I started to pray. The spirits showed me what to say. When I was done, I still felt the same and just a little disappointed. We left for the hospital. The closest hospital to us was York-Central in Richmond Hill, Ontario.

After a few ex-rays the doctor returned to where I was laying on a gurney in the hallway, it was very busy that night. All the emergency rooms were full. He said that I was pretty sick and must be in a lot of pain. I replied that I'd seen better days. Ironically, he had found three stones in my gall bladder. I would have to have surgery to remove them. I say ironically because here I was making a living and supporting my family with small stones and it was small stones also causing me a problem. Or were they in fact making me slow down? Were they bringing me the message that I needed to rest and recuperate? Sometimes it's very hard to know why things happen. If this hadn't happened to slow me down would something more serious have happened to me?

Then he told me how much it was going to cost per day. That almost gave me a heart attack! Turning I looked at my wife. She had a very worried look on her face. I started to get up as I asked for my clothes. There was no way I could afford it, I told him. He said to get back in bed, then he whispered in my ear that I couldn't be refused treatment so not to worry about it. After the doctor left, Melody asked me what he had said. When I told her, there was an immediate change in her look and attitude. She said not to worry this was her country and they wouldn't let us down, besides she said, "the Great Spirit is watching over us."

I was kept in the hospital for several days. They were waiting for the infection to go down before they could operate on me. During the wait I caught pneumonia and was sicker yet. On the fourth morning I woke up feeling so sick, it took me several hours to realize I no longer had the abdominal pain.

A week later I was sent home to get over the infection of the pneumonia. Before I went home they did another ex-ray. Then they did a cat scan. My doctor was simply amazed he couldn't find the stones in my gall bladder. He didn't know what had happened. They had monitored me so well, he said I hadn't passed them. If I had, I would have known it. I've heard that it's pretty painful.

He said that all he could find was something that looked like sludge. As though the stones had dissolved. Was the Stone People Medicine working for me? They had healed me and I felt great. In trying to explain to the doctor about our ways, it went over his head. Perhaps he wasn't ready to learn other ways. I felt sorry for him.

As it turned out, I never had surgery. In fact, I never had to go back to the hospital. I've given what happened a lot of thought since then and I've come to the conclusion that both the doctor and I had lessons to learn through my experience. My lesson was to believe in the power of the stones and have confidence in myself. His was to learn there are other alternative forms of medicine and it's there for all to use. He missed the whole thing.

3. Different ways stones are used today.

Some consider certain stones too common to acknowledge. That's where native people differ from the rest of the world. Most world people have advanced so much scientifically or maybe regressed, that they have forgotten the importance of nature. They have forgotten the importance of asking the oldest entity on this earth for advice and counsel.

The Plains tribes have the Sweat Lodge ceremony. It is the grandfather of all ceremonies. No other ceremony is conducted without the Sweat Lodge first taking place. The participants in a Sweat Lodge ceremony use large, hot rocks preheated in a fire pit. We believe that the Grandfather's breath (the steam) brings you a spiritual cleansing inside and out, for whatever ceremony or path that you are seeking at the time.

Lets look at one stone in particular, the crystal. I'm talking about the crystals because I like them and I believe in their power. I want to emphasize that native people didn't look at crystals as anything special. No more than any other stone created by the Great Spirit. Many ask what is so special about crystals. It has properties unlike any other stone. It has the ability to amplify energy very much like our bodies. We eat food and convert it into energy. The crystal on the other hand absorbs electrical impulses or spiritual energy and amplifies them. Spiritual energy you ask? Prayers, hopes, needs, wishes, they are all a form of spiritual supplication and energy. If spiritual energy generated by prayer is not effective then why do we pray? Why do we bother with all we do for spiritual fulfillment?

A crystal has the capability to amplify a radio signal or electrical impulse sent to it, as it rides in a scientific contraption called a satellite.

It can do that and then redirect it in another direction. It also has the capability to receive spiritual energy. By the way spirits and radio signals or impulses are all invisible yet they both exist. Most important is that they both work.

Advanced scientific minds think that the computers have all the answers! Well even computers need a slice of quartz crystal in the microchip. Why do you think that quartz watches can run so long on those tiny batteries? The reason is that the quartz in the watch amplifies the energy of the battery giving it a longer life. Then there's the satellite out in space. Because of the quartz crystals, it can receive solar energy and convert it to usable energy. The energy can operate the equipment on board for months and even years at a time. Also it can receive impulses or signals from earth, amplify them and send them back to different locations on earth.

This technology is possible only because we have the quartz crystals. The very laptop computer screen I'm typing this book into is made of liquid crystals. Man has learned to duplicate crystals but they have had to follow the same formula that nature uses. Where did that knowledge come from? Could that knowledge have come to the inventor from the stones themselves? He must have been ready and open to receive or he wouldn't have received that idea.

Many forget it was a person like themselves who put that information into the computer. That is another difference between us. Many native people have not forgotten where we came from. We haven't forgotten where wisdom waits. Where we as individuals can access all this knowledge and information.

It takes a long time to gain knowledge and wisdom. If it takes us humans fifteen to twenty years to get a good education, can you imagine the vast amounts of knowledge stones have accumulated in their billions of years of existence? So many things happened while the stones were forming. So many people, animals, insects walked or flew by the stones. Each leaving a small residue of itself on the stone. Each little bit of residue turning into another tiny bit of knowledge ingrained within the molecules of the stone. All that accumulation of bits of information comes to us as usable knowledge.

We've talked about the practical uses of stones and the religious beliefs. There is an increasing fascination with stones in today's movie business. Just look at a small sample of recent movies that feature a stone as the main plot, or some aspect of the story. Movies such as, "The Dark Crystal," "Superman," "Romancing the Stone," "Sword in the Stone," "Indiana Jones and the Temple of Doom." Even as Pocahontas sings, "Colors of the Wind" at the beginning of the song, she places her hand on a large stone and says, "Everything has a spirit, has a name." The stone lights up under her hand, as though happy for the recognition.

In fact, one of our Stone People Medicine, the Snake, was used in an episode of "Kung Fu the Legend Continues." David Carradine's character, Kane used our stone as a method of helping save a young girl's life. He told her to speak through the stone to call him and he would come to help her. The popularity of these films shows the interest people have in stones, their credibility and their mystical properties.

The most primitive men, used stones

to throw, made arrowheads, beads and weapons. While also using stones to build shelters, men's lives have always been in constant relationships with stones one way or another. We have placed high values on some of them like diamonds, emeralds and rubies, yet others we just kick out of the way.

What about Stone Henge - who really knows where these phenomenal stone monoliths came from. Was it a place for sacrifices? A blessed and holy place? Or was it just a popular marketplace? Are people drawn there because the stone formations have knowledge to give to those open to receive? There are those who go through a great deal of trouble in Ireland to kiss the Blarney Stone. Why? There are legends, but, is that all there is to the story?

Easter Island is another stone mystery. How did those giant stone statues arrive? Who carved them and for what reason? Were they considered stones of knowledge? Were they given human like features because of the wisdom they offered?

Even more intriguing are the stone pyramids of Egypt, no one knows why they were built or how. All archaeologists can do, is speculate. How about the pyramids of the Aztecs and the Toltecs in Mexico? The pyramids were built of stone. Was it because of the spiritual nature of stone and the guidance received by those worshipping on the pyramids? Also the huge Dream Stone in Australia, used by the aborigine people to record all their history. The Wailing Wall in Jerusalem is a stone wall used to place prayers within the stones. People believe that this will take your prayers directly to God.

What about the people in Africa? There's one tribe of people that go to a spiritual place and quarry a special stone. They crush it to a fine powder, then wet and roll it into oblong pieces that look like dough. Then with contentment on their faces, they sit and eat it as though it were candy.

Even the Plains people used stones to hold down the edge of their tepees during inclement weather and it was also done with ceremony. The enormous Stone Medicine Wheel in Wyoming that can only be seen from the sky is another example. For thousands of years, the Medicine Wheel was used by native people for seeking direction, wisdom from the stones and guidance from the spirits. To this day the Medicine Wheel (circle) remains as the most powerful symbol available.

The list goes on and on, there are too many to list in this book. However the theme is the same, stones have proven to be a significant and largely spiritual influence on the world from yesterday and today.

All these stone forms have left us all baffled and fascinated. From cliff dwellings to diamonds, man has surrounded himself with stones since the beginning of time. Many of us don't realize where this knowledge, wisdom and new ideas comes from. Its time to give credit where credit is due.

SECTION II
Spirit Animals/Figures

This section will reveal each Stone People Medicine animals/figures and their relationship to us humans. Their behavior, characteristics and how this ties in spiritually with the medicine they offer you, will be shown. There are many different animals to use, however these are the animals given to me in dreams.

Why have the spirit of animals become known as our protectors, guides and advisors? I believe the reason the creator appointed the animal spirits to help humans is, they are without prejudice or egos. They see life through very different and simple eyes compared to us. Animals use only what is necessary for surviving. The guidance they offer is of the purist form.

Although the description of how each animal helps you is on the card inside the bag with the stone, within this book you'll find a more detailed explanation on the different figures. As you read about each one, you'll find you have a heartfelt attraction for one figure, over the others. I have found that most times it's better to go with your first choice. Your first choice is your intuition, after that your logic kicks in and talks you out of the best choice for yourself. It's important that you read about all of them to find out which one if your spirit helper. If you don't feel a strong attraction to any one figure, close your eyes and let the stone come to you. Whatever figure is on the stone, invariably it will be what you need in your life.

Then we have the human type spirits. They are here to show us the way through the difficult times in our lives. To help us with emotional problems of the heart. When we need them, the old spirits are always willing to step forward to help us. They come to us with different names and seem to always come to us in dreams. I believe they are old spirits that have finally reached their ultimate goal of spiritual perfection. Now one of their spiritual duties is helping us find our paths to their spiritual elevation. Other ways the spirits help us, is showing us how to pray and show respect to the Great Spirit. They bring us what we need to cope with our emotional lives, and give guidance to our minds. I say they help us with our minds because our mind is the most powerful part of our body. Our mind can help us do things beyond our wildest dreams. That's where the Stone People Medicine comes in. As powerful as the mind is, it is worthless without knowledge and guidance. The power and knowledge to direct the mind is supplied by the prayer and the stones.

Human type spirits always give themselves either masculine or feminine names, depending on who is asking for help. The reason I say they give themselves these names, is that in their world there is no difference. There are no males or females only the spirits. The spirits come to us in the form that we will be the most comfortable with and will accept the help without hesitation. When these spirits lived as we do now, they were willing to suffer for others. They were willing to offer themselves in sacrifice so that others could live better. Therefore they reached the level that allows them to help others on a permanent basis.

Although the human spirits demand a complete book of their own, the main thing that we are concerned with is the animal spirits. I'll discuss the ways that they can help us. I believe that they are our life guides.

The Great Spirit gave us the animal spirits, so we could help ourselves. Animal spirits help us with our life guidance and the stones bring us the wisdom we need. It truly works. All you have to do is believe in it.

Here are some testimonials of how the Stone People Medicine have helped people that believed in them.

I was at a gem and mineral show in Denver, Colorado a few years ago, when a young man and his wife stopped to talk to me. They were very interested in the Stone People Medicine. I explained about the different ways the stones could help people using them. When he heard me talk about how Kokopelli was the bringer of babies, he got really interested. He asked if it would help them. They had been trying to conceive for six years without success. I told him that Kokopelli could be asked to help and he would. I told them to put the stone under their pillow and wait for results.

Approximately six months later I saw him again at another show in Tucson, Arizona. When he saw me from a distance of about twenty feet he yelled happily, "Manny, it works, we're four months pregnant!" Since then I've seen him, his wife and a beautiful little baby boy. They are as thoroughly convinced as I am that the stones do work.

This next story is also one that borders on the incredible.

A lady in a Midwestern state is a very good customer of mine. She has a store with all top quality Native American crafts. One spring when everyone is concerned about paying their taxes, she found herself in the same situation. Her accountant told her she owed the government three thousand, five hundred dollars. Spring is her worst time of the year, business wise, she pointed out.

While at her store where she carries all the Stone People Medicine, she reached into the basket and pulled the Buffalo . In sheer desperation she talked to the Buffalo Medicine. She told it she needed thirty-five-hundred dollars by Monday. This was Friday morning. She told me that she really didn't believe in them, but she was desperate.

On Saturday morning when she got to the store there were people waiting for her to open. The morning got very busy. The store was jumping with people. They were busy buying this and that. There seemed to be a special energy in the air. It takes a lot of sales for any store to have a big day. It happened here when it was needed. By early that afternoon she had exactly thirty five-hundred dollars in the till. Business died down after that. She also told me that she has had need of help two or three times since then and she has never been let down.

This story is one that really touched my heart. I was at a Native arts & crafts show in the little town of San Juan Bautista, California. A young man came by my booth. After I explained the different stones he decided to take a Bear Medicine to a sister. He didn't tell me why he was getting it.

Several months later I was doing another Native show in the same place and town. The guy that had bought the Bear Medicine stone came looking for me. He had a smile on his face as he happily shook my hand. Then he told me the story of why he had returned to see me. His sister had been in a lot of pain. They had found out she had cancer. After she received the Bear Stone People Medicine her pain started going away.

Day after day she had less and less pain. By the time he came to see me the second time they had received the good news that the cancer was in remission. So he wanted more stones for other people.

Was it coincidence or were these seeming miracles going to happen anyway? Only the Great Spirit knows, but I feel good about what has happened. I have faith and confidence in the Stone People Medicine.

One final little story to show you how Stones use us as transportation to reach the person, they need to get to.

While on a drive in northern California, we got to the beach and stopped. We walked on the beach looking for shells. I saw a beautiful stone. It was dark green, almost black. Although larger than I wanted to carry, I was compelled to pick it up and take it home.

We were camping at the K.O.A. Campground in San Juan Bautista. After we got back, I showed it to a friend of mine asking what it was. He replied it was top quality serpentine. I kept it for a few days. When we were getting ready to leave to go east, I told my wife that I was going to leave the stone there at the campground. I can't explain what happened next.

Without anyone or anything touching the stone, it suddenly rolled off the table. Before I could move out of the way it had already hit me. Here's the odd thing. When something falls the law of gravity says that it will fall straight down to the floor. The stone should have landed on my toes. It didn't do what it was supposed to. I don't know why, but it hit my shin bone and left a bruise about the size of an egg. It was painful for three weeks.

So after it did that to me I took the hint that it didn't want to be left behind. So we took the stone with us. Before we left, our friends were over to see us again. Looking at the stone again our friend said, "Manny there's a face on this stone." I looked at it and sure enough there was a face silhouette on it. It was a fracture in the stone but it was an almost perfect profile.

When we got to South Bend, Indiana the next month to do a show, a young woman walked in and came straight to our table. She had a postcard with my picture on it. It had been given to her by a friend. We had sent a lot of them to people on our mailing list. Two days before that, she had drawn my face, although she had never heard of me or seen me. As an artist, all she had ever been able to draw was half a face and she does a beautiful job of it. When I showed her the stone with the profile on it, she completely lost it, and started crying uncontrollably. I didn't know what to do, and never expected a reaction like this. Perhaps the energy of the stone and the silhouette on it really moved her emotionally and spiritually. So I gave it to her. I knew then the stone had used me to transport it from the beach in California to whom it belonged, this woman in Indiana. Perhaps in time the stone will help her to complete her pictures.

There are many more stories like this and maybe someday I'll put them in a book of short stories about how stones helped people.

Spider Medicine

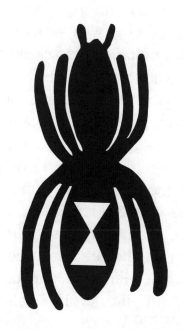

With its endless patterns and combinations in its web, Spider has become the Symbol of infinity, it brings to you limitless possibilities. Mystic Medicine weaves its way into your life, helping you see with your psychic intuition. Spider medicine reminds you to put your thoughts to paper and write. Clearing your head of all the cobwebs building up inside to make room for fresh creativity, and clean thoughts. Communication improves with Spider's help.

If there is any doubt as to the power of Spider medicine, think about this. Why is the largest communication network in the world called the "World Wide Web?" Use the web in Spider medicine to help yourself without reservations. This medicine helps you remember that there's always options in life.

Many species have eight eyes. This physical characteristic can be used to help you spot opportunities coming to you from any direction. This medicine also helps in making decisions about career choices.

Spider medicine helps you to be resilient to change, and adapt to new life situations quickly. Spider medicine enables you to be diverse and better equipped to cope in the changing times coming for all of us.

Spider may be small, yet it is a powerful insect, honored by some native societies as a being of mystical powers. It can help the persons drawn to it with the power of manifestation and creating special situations.

What you can expect from Spider medicine:

* Limitless possibilities

* Psychic intuition

* Life options

* Career choices

* Manifestation

Turtle Medicine

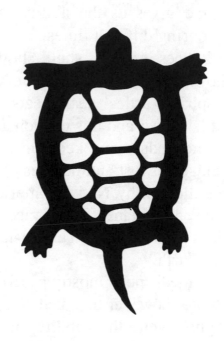

Turtle is patient, determined and strong. Turtle Medicine teaches us patience with ourselves and others; determination to finish whatever we start; and gives us the ability to be strong during difficult times.

Turtle goes inside its shell, showing you how to reflect and improve your inner spirit. Turtles' heart beats days after it has died, and this medicine can help us to endure and keep on living after all seems lost and hopeless.

Once thought by Native Americans to be the entire planet, Turtle medicine brings us the strength of Turtle Island - Mother Earth.

Turtle medicine is mostly passive in its defense, however this medicine can also give you the ability to be aggressive and protect yourself from those that would take advantage of you. Once a turtle gets a hold of something, because its jaws are so powerful, unless it releases by choice, death is the only other way to make it let go. This medicine can give you the stubbornness to have your way in whatever you choose.

Due to its longevity, Turtle medicine shows us that you can endure without being aggressive in your defense. Turtles have been around this earth millions of years. They are passive in their defense, and sluggish in their movements. However, they have endured the test of time, and perhaps we can all learn a lesson from the medicine they offer.

Though it moves very slowly, it is determined to reach its chosen destination. With Turtle medicine you can also have the same attributes and are able to apply them to everyday life. Like the Turtle, be strong and persistent in your quest.

What you can expect from Turtle medicine:

* Determination

* Strength

* Endurance

* Patience

Snake Medicine

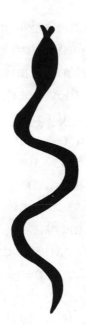

Just like a snake sheds its skin to let go of the old and make room for new growth, Snake medicine helps you release your old life or old habits and start anew.

It gives you the wisdom and power to change negative thoughts. Snakes have well-developed muscles and only eat as much as they need. You can ask Snake to help you tone your body and keep you from over indulging. Like the Snake scents the air with its tongue, you can also learn to feel if good or bad is coming towards you and act accordingly.

Snakes are called cold blooded animals, and they spend a lot of time seeking warmth, so this medicine will help you bring love and warmth into others' hearts.

Snake has the ability to camouflage

itself, to protect it from danger. You also can benefit from this trait and keep your feelings hidden. This will keep you from allowing yourself to be vulnerable.

Snake is the symbol of life, death, rebirth, the afterlife and sacred knowledge (Garden of Eden). There was an ancient snake cult in Egypt, and it is believed that circumcision may have originated from that, to emulate the snake shedding its skin.

When it comes to supplying energy and determination to humans, Snake medicine is unsurpassed in strength for starting new endeavors, lives or even careers. Snake medicine enables you to change your life when the one you have is impossible.

What you can expect from Snake medicine:

* Help release the old (relationships-problems)

* Life, career

* Power to change negative thoughts

* Strong determination

Man-in-the-Maze Medicine

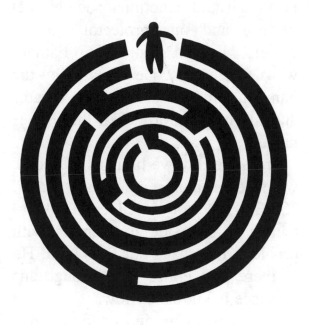

"Se-Eh-Ha" is your personal spirit guide through life. The maze signifies our world, with all the twists and turns of life. Also, could be called your native guardian angel. "Older Brother" is our spiritual, emotional and physical balance and our protector. In the center, "E-Thoi" our "Sun Father" waits to bless us. He takes us by the hand and introduces us to the creator and the next world when this life is passed.

From the day we humans are born, we face problems on a daily basis. "Se-Eh-Ha", our "Older Brother" comes to our side to help us with problems that make our lives hard. He is there our entire life, though his presence is known by few.

We have all experienced times when we have gotten ourselves into what we think is a major problem. Suddenly, without any effort from us, except the worry and lost sleep, the problem we thought was so big, disappears. That's when "Se-Eh-Ha" has stepped in to help one of his charges.

Treat the Man-in-the-Maze with respect and help is always yours.

What you can expect from Man-in-the-Maze Medicine:

* Your own Native Guardian Angel

* Protection from problems

* Balance

* Guidance

Kokopelli Medicine

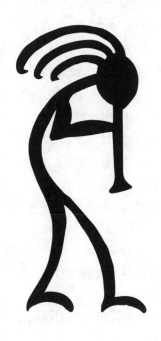

Kokopelli was respected by all the tribes that knew of him, and was thought to bring good luck to all that received him. Each village he visited gave him the finest gifts. He in turn would give the gifts to the next village he visited. Consequently he gave only the best gifts. It gave him the reputation of being a very generous man. This medicine teaches us to only give the very best of ourselves. We must also be willing to receive the best from others, keeping your life in balance. When Kokopelli was in the village everyone celebrated. He brought happiness and harmony to homes.

Sometimes Kokopelli was thought of as the one who brought babies. Often he helped couples that were infertile, to finally experience the joys of parenthood. The magic from his flute playing can stimulate creativity and helps dreams come true.

When it was found out that Kokopelli was on his way the village elders would select a willing girl to spend the night with him. It was considered an honor for him to accept her. If she conceived a child during their union, the girl, her child and her family were treated like royalty from that time on.

Though he was a mortal man, the good he imparted (life counseling, spiritual guidance, important news) through so many years he became like a god! He was so respected (his advice almost always proved to be correct) that people started chipping his image on stones and cave walls.

Kokopelli traveled far and wide. His

image has been found from the Yucatan Peninsula in Mexico to as far north as New Mexico.

Many of the petroglyphs portrayed him with his erect penis. When the Spanish Christians arrived they noticed the high esteem Kokopelli was held, they immediately started intervening on how Kokopelli was painted. Though the Spanish couldn't stop the honoring, painting and respect of this image, they did succeed in getting the natives to change the pictures to one of a man without his manhood. Lately I've seen some artists beginning to portray him, complete with his manhood, as proud as ever.

If you need help in being creative in your life Kokopelli is the one for you. He helps writers, sculptors, artists (clay, paint, glass), and helps you create things of beauty. Respect what he represents and you will be justly compensated. If you want to begin something new in the arts or writing etc, he can help immensely.

What you can expect from Kokopelli medicine:

* Fertility

* Creativity in the arts

* Sexuality

* Inspiration

Eagle Medicine

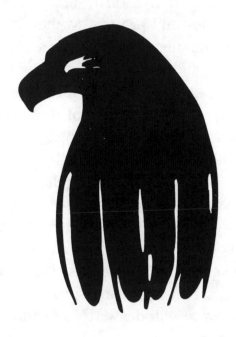

If the Eagle comes to you or you choose it, you have a powerful commitment to prayer. The Eagle is the highest flying bird, and carries your wishes and prayers to the Great Spirit to be answered. This warrior's bird reminds you to reach for higher goals and know you can achieve them.

Always a symbol of warrior societies, the strength and protection from the Eagle can be used in your favor. Let the Eagle spirit help you fight your battles, and protect you from your enemies. Eagle medicine gives you the ability to look at yourself with eagle eyes and assess what you truly need materially and spiritually. It can help you withdraw from everyday interruptions and to focus on what needs to be accomplished to make your life better.

The Eagle is also represented as a Thunderbird. It is believed that the Thunderbird controls lightning, storms and thunder. Some cultures believed if a Lightning Bird strikes at a certain spot, the stones found there are really the eggs of the Eagle or Lightning Bird. The Thunderbird is also considered to be the guardian of the heavens. Thunderclaps are believed to be the flaps of eagles' wings, and lightning is the eagle eye flashing.

The Eagle is the most important member of the animal world to the Native Americans. Every part of the eagle is sacred, particularly the feathers. When the Eagle passes into the spirit world, it leaves its body behind to help native people. We use the head on top of a sacred staff. It in essence becomes our flag and something to follow.

Many traditional dancers use its talons on personal dance staffs. They also represent that we are willing to defend our families and spiritual beliefs. The Eagle bone whistle that comes from the wing, makes the sound of the Eagle calling its mate. This same sound carries our prayers to the Great Spirit.

The Eagle feathers are so important to native people that a man had to earn the right to wear one through great accomplishments. Men earned them on the battlefield, through participation in the Sundance, and undergoing the piercing ceremony. Even today, both men and women are still awarded Eagle feathers for completing deeds of great accomplishments. They can consist of finishing High School, completing College, University or by serving in the military forces. The Eagle feathers to this day continue to be sacred to our people. Its a big honor to receive one, they are always given in ceremony.

During any social gathering or ceremony, such as a pow wow or demonstration dances, if an eagle feather falls from any dancer's outfit, everything comes to a complete standstill. That feather symbolizes a fallen warrior. That warrior and feather are to be respected and treated in a sacred way. A ceremony for the fallen feather is done, generally with four veterans that are called forward to perform the ceremony. It cannot just be picked up. After the ceremony is finished, the feather is picked up and placed on a drum. The owner of the feather must claim his/her feather, and honor with a monetary gift, each and every one involved in the ceremony.

It is also a federal law in the United States, it carries a heavy penalty of jail and large fines, to sell any part of an eagle. Only Native Americans can have Eagle feathers in their possession, but never for sale.

The majesty of the Eagle is yours when you need it. Its devotion to others, the courage to accomplish and defend what is yours, the pride in yourself as a person is all covered by that grand majesty. The Great Spirit always listens to the Eagle's voice.

What you can expect from Eagle Medicine:

* Prayers answered

* Achieving higher goals

* Self-assessment

* Pride and courage

Bear Medicine

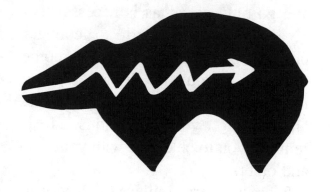

Bear medicine gives you the ability to go as far as you need, to accomplish things that you might have thought were completely out of your reach. Yet at the same time, it brings you the wisdom to take only what you need, and go only as far as is necessary. It gives you the strength to conquer physical problems, and to overcome obstacles in your life. It can help you in your dreams, to recall them and find answers to your questions. Bear reminds you to be gentle with yourself, and others.

Bears are very similar in behavior to humans. They walk upright on two legs. They are nurturing toward their young. Bears build up their winter coats to protect themselves. Bear medicine gives you the ability to cover yourself with strength and pride.

For those who have not made their mark in life, Bear medicine helps you establish your territory, realize your gifts and gives you the strength to use your gifts and abilities to advance yourself.

Bears are solitary creatures by nature. Bear medicine helps us when we are alone, learn to enjoy our own company and become self reliant. With the many distractions life has to offer, solitude helps us get our thoughts, and minds together to stay in balance.

Bear gives you the ability to find your way back into the life of someone you may have lost in the past. If you've neglected a gift or creative ability you have, Bear helps you retrieve that loss and use it again.

Bear helps you to cover your feelings, when and if you are being pressured to reveal personal thoughts. If you are being annoyed by someone, Bear teaches you how to avoid uncomfortable situations.

Bear medicine can help bring back a sense of order into your life, when its chaotic and confusing.

Many Native people use Bear spirit to help remove illness from anyone that needs that help. Bear medicine can give a person the strength to overcome any illness, mental, spiritual or physical.

Being the largest and most powerful animal in North America, its medicine is equal in size when it comes to help us.

What you can expect from Bear Medicine:

* Spiritual strength

* Conquer physical problems

* Be self-reliant

* Self advancement

Buffalo Medicine

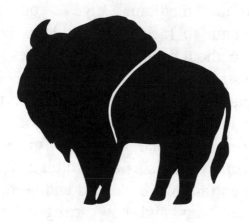

Good luck medicine. Buffalo means abundance in all aspects of life, love, health, happiness and wealth. Count on many things coming your way and be grateful for all it brings to you. Buffalo medicine gives you the strength to face your problems head on, without backing down. It gives you the strength during hard times.

Native Americans used every part of the buffalo. The flesh for food, the bones for tools, the hides for tepee covers, moccasins and clothing. Even the entrails were cleaned and used for water bags and bow strings. Dried Buffalo meat mixed with berries and grease (pemmican) made excellent high protein food. It kept the members of the village well fed while on the move. Always grateful for all the buffalo brings to them, Native

Americans had elaborate ceremonies before and after a buffalo hunt. The Buffalo is also very important in the Sundance ceremony. They would show respect for the buffalo spirit for bringing them such abundance. Buffalo shows us not to be wasteful and to use our gifts wisely.

People who tend to let others walk all over them, can use the Buffalo medicine to help them speak up for themselves and not simply take whatever others dish out.

Both male and female buffalo have horns. This medicine allows you to protect yourself from anything or anyone that tries to harm you.

Buffalo medicine gives you the ability to take energy, store it and call on it whenever you need it. Giving you the strength to nourish yourself spiritually, emotionally and physically.

When Buffalo medicine comes to you, treat it with respect and all it has to offer will be yours.

What you can expect from Buffalo medicine:

* Good Luck

* Abundance

* Strength

* Teaches us not to be wasteful

Wolf Medicine

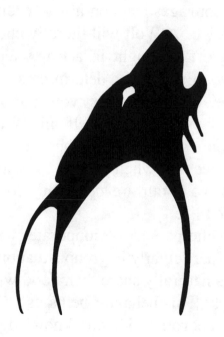

Wolf medicine helps you to become dynamic and outgoing. Wolf is a teacher. It helps us to learn and communicate that knowledge to others and encourages us open up to receive knowledge. A Wolf will literally chew his leg off if caught in a trap. Wolf gives you the will and determination to be free of restrictions you put on yourself or find yourself in. Wolf medicine shows you when to be aggressive and when to hold back and be passive, both are necessary for a balanced life.

Wolf helps us to cooperate with others, particularly in group situations. Wolves naturally share their food with the pack. This behavior helps us to be more generous with our knowledge, time and material things.

Like the Wolf's determination to

keep itself on track to find its prey, even at long distances, his medicine also helps you stick with what you want to accomplish. Keep on and don't give up on your desires, no matter how long it takes to achieve your goals.

Wolves live in packs or tribes. They choose a leader and have followers. This trait can help you realize when its time to lead and when its time to follow. Similar to the old saying, "The true teacher is also always a good student."

Their keen sense of smell and hearing gives them an alertness that we can use to protect us. Wolf medicine can help you sense bad things coming your way. Listen to those feelings as you hold Wolf medicine.

Wolf medicine will help you realize the goal you are reaching for is within the realm of possibilities for you. The same way a Wolf will not chase anything to eat that uses up more energy getting it, than it can replace.

When Wolf medicine comes to you, treat it with respect and it will repay you in ways you never dreamed. Let the Wolf medicine bring you the knowledge you need to advance not only intellectually but also with stealth and cunning.

Wolf medicine is for the person always yearning to learn and yet willing to teach. Also for special people who are willing to share his/her expertise and knowledge.

What you can expect from Wolf Medicine:

* Ability to learn and teach easily

* Communicate

* Strong determination

* To be thoughtful of others

Otter Medicine

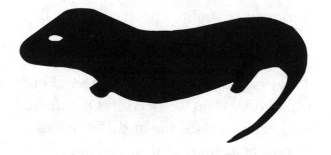

Otter is known as Woman Medicine. It gives you clean and powerful energy for creativity and manifestation. Otter teaches you to be resourceful and remember you can endure and be stronger than you think.

Otter teaches us to play and not take life too seriously. We have become too seriously caught up in day to day living. Playing and enjoying what life has to offer has become secondary. Otter medicine brings back a bit of our childhood when we need it. Otter helps us keep our chin up in difficult times and to be resourceful in finding things we need.

Because Otter moves equally fast on any terrain, this medicine enables you to reach your destination in life, regardless of the path you have chosen.

Although Otters are cute and seemingly playful, people getting too close to them can cause it to become very ferocious and protective. If you have chosen the Otter it can bring you these same qualities. Being ferocious in pursuing love, opportunities or any other things you desire. Treat the Otter with respect and you will receive strong energy in return.

What to expect from Otter Medicine:

* Powerful energy

* Power of manifestation

* Resourcefulness

* Protectiveness

SECTION III

Using Stone People Medicine

1. Daily uses to help yourself

There are several ways to use the Stone People Medicine. I'll outline the different ways that I know on how to use them. Then after you start using them, you might find other ways to use the stones. Our minds, thoughts and inventiveness are our only limitations when it comes to using the Stone People Medicine.

One way to use the stones is for self-help. Find and pick the animal/stone that you like best. This way you only have one stone and can focus all your energy on that aspect of your life. You might find that you need one, two or maybe three stones. That's fine because we're all human and need help in different areas of our lives. Then there is some of you that will want to have them all. One reason having the entire set of stones is important, is you can draw a different stone, with eyes closed, each day for guidance. This allows your personal energy or intuition to bring you the stone you need for that day. It's important that you allow that stone and spirit animal to help you. If you use this method of picking your stone for the day, you'll find, more often than not, it will actually be what you needed. Even if it isn't a conscious reason, it most certainly will be helpful on an unconscious level.

When choosing a stone, ask yourself which of the little figures appeals to you. Find out what area of your life you need the most help in.

You might find times in your life that you're angry, upset, confused, financially embarrassed, or depressed. All those terrible things that happen to humans. Everyone goes through these feelings one time or another. This is where Stone People Medicine can help. There's a stone or figure that can help you in any way you might need. For example you find that you need help with your health, the Bear Medicine would be the stone to help you. If you're an artist, writer or carver, there is times your mind goes blank. It seems that ideas won't come to you no matter what you do. When this happens, the stone with Kokopelli on it is the one for you.

He is the one that brings inspiration

to people whether they are creative or not. It's up to you to find what you need.

If you don't feel an attraction to any of the figures then you must allow the stone to call or talk to you. The way to do this is to close your eyes, take a deep breath and calm yourself. Put all the stones you have in front of you. Slowly run your hands back and forth over them until one feels good to you or until you choose one.

One way to use the stones is, by holding it in your hand. *You do not pray to the stone, you only hold it while you pray.* For example: if you choose Wolf medicine, because you wish to learn something, hold it in your hand. You can ask out loud, "I need help in finding the answer to this question I've got."   Then ask the question. It's as simple as that. You can use any of the Stone People Medicine as simply as that. Be direct, ask what you want to know or for the help you need. Don't ever let the word greed, hold you back from asking for what you need or want. The Spirits don't recognize that word. It was probably invented by a person that was jealous of someone having more than they did.

Don't be impatient, wait for an answer. It will come to you. Sometimes the answer is almost immediate, sometimes it's an hour, a day or longer, but Stones and spirit animals do bring answers and guidance.

Another reason you may want to have the entire set is to use them to help others. However, this can only be effective if you've learned to help yourself first, and have learned to use the stones properly. By this I mean that you have to learn how to open your mind up to be able to receive the messages brought to you by the spirits and the stones. That's the reason the stones and pictures of the spirits are together. The guidance they bring is very powerful. And the only way that you can get good and proficient in using the stones is by practicing over and over. Listen with your mind and your heart.

2. Ways to help others

When you're confident working with the Stone People Medicine and can clearly interpret what they bring you, then you're ready to help others. Here's how you can help them. This is the way I do it. Sit them down with a small table between you. I lay the stones face down in front of the person I'm helping. Help them relax with good clean spiritual conversation. Then with their eyes closed ask them to pick five or seven stones depending on how detailed a reading they want.

As with all other types of helping methods the sequence the stones are picked is very important. The same stone picked by a different person could have a totally different meaning. Before I attempt to interpret the stones for people I always ask the spirits for their help, guidance and for the wisdom to interpret the stones wisely, with a prayer.

When helping others, I do what I call a mini reading/interpretation ten to fifteen minutes long. Also I do a full reading/interpretation that lasts twenty-five to thirty minutes. Sometimes, I do longer readings on special requests.

3. Sample layouts for interpretations

One layout I do is called **The Five Directions**. As the person pulls five stones and hands them to me, I place them in what I call the five directions. The first stone is to the persons left. It symbolizes the **EAST** direction. Always place yourself in the south direction making the other person sitting at the north direction. Stone number two is placed in front of you and is the **SOUTH** direction. The third stone is placed to their right and the **WEST** direction. Stone number four is placed in front of them and is the **NORTH** direction stone. The fifth and last stone is placed in the center making it the **INNER** direction or their spirit stone and very important. This is the stone and spirit animal that is going to show direction.

No matter where you are sitting, just assume that it's always the south position, and the person getting the reading sits in the north position. The stones are kept face down the entire time. Interpret them one at a time as they are turned over. Always begin with the first stone, the EAST direction one. Then go on to the SOUTH, WEST, NORTH and finally the center or INNER direction. As shown in the diagram.

FIVE DIRECTIONS LAYOUT

other person

N

W   I   E

S

you

Another layout I use is called **The Seven Stone Mound**, and the order of the stones is as follows: As the person picks out the stones one at a time, place the first one the **EAST** direction to their left. Then the next three, **SOUTH**, then **WEST**, and the **NORTH** direction, toward their right, in a straight line with the first one. The fifth stone the **ABOVE** direction and the sixth one is the **BELOW** direction are above the first four, from their left to right. The final stone, the INNER direction is placed above the others, in the center. Again, the stones are kept face down until you're ready to start interpreting them. You should start with the first one, then on through to the top one. That one I believe is that persons direction stone and very important. See the diagram.

SEVEN STONE MOUND

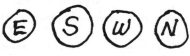

YOU

Ⓘ

Ⓐ   Ⓑ

Ⓔ Ⓢ Ⓦ Ⓝ

Other Person

Interpret them as before. Listen to your heart. Listen to the Spirits and tell the person seeking your help what the stones bring you. I never make any life and death comments. You don't want to plant a seed and cause anything to happen because they expect it. The Great Spirit guides me to tell them about other things that are important. I try to give as positive an interpretation as I possibly can or I feel as though I'm not doing my job or what I'm being paid to do.

If you're planning to help people in a professional way it's always good to have two complete sets of the stones. This way it gives their energy or inner feelings more choices to pick from. If two of the same spirit animals are picked that could mean their needs are very high in that area. Also any figure chosen means a different thing, depending on the direction it is chosen in. See the explanation of each figure in each direction, to follow these layouts.

Turn over the stones in the same sequence as placed and interpret them to the best of your ability. One very important point that you must know is every stone has two or more ways to interpret it. As the person doing the reading its up to you to find the information that belongs to the person in front of you. Remember, listen to the Spirit Animals and the stones. They will bring you all you need to tell that person. Be sincere, don't try to make things up. Remember, as you work with these stones you will be receiving guidance for these people. They will believe what you say, that is the reason they have come to you. Speak only the truth. Sincerity and truth are most important. Your words may change their lives. It's very important you use these stones in a good way. If the truth is going to hurt them, you might try to use different words to prevent that hurt. The road we choose to help others is a very delicate one and with a fine edge. You have the power to either help immensely or you could to a lot of damage to peoples hearts and minds. Walk the edge with extreme care and with a warm and loving heart. Remember every time you help someone, the spirits will repay you by bringing more good things into your life.

4. The Seven Directions Quick Reference Guide

The following seven pages contain a quick reference guide, helping you in your interpretations, using the five and seven direction layout. It is up to you to interpret the combinations of stones with the direction that falls in sequence. This is just a guide, once you are in tune with the stones, your interpretations may vary from this guide.

The East Direction is where the sun rises every morning, bringing the whole world new life and us our daily blessings.

Spider: Limitless possibilities, psychic intuition, career choices

Turtle: Patience, endurance in difficult times, determination

Snake: New life, releasing the old, power to change

Man-in-the-Maze: Spiritual, emotional, physical balance, guidance

Kokopelli: Inspiration, creativity, fertility, sexuality

Eagle: Prayers answered, pride and courage, self-assessment

Bear: Strength, courage, overcome physical problems, self-reliance

Buffalo: Abundance, face problems head on, good luck

Wolf: Teacher medicine, determination, communication

Otter: Powerful energy, creativity, manifestation, resourcefulness

The South Direction is where the warm winds come from to bring an end to the coldness of winter and new life to all.

Spider: Limitless possibilities, psychic intuition, career choices

Turtle: Patience, endurance in difficult times, determination

Snake: New life, releasing the old, power to change

Man-in-the-Maze: Spiritual, emotional, physical balance, guidance

Kokopelli: Inspiration, creativity, fertility, sexuality

Eagle: Prayers answered, pride and courage, self-assessment

Bear: Strength, courage, overcome physical problems, self-reliance

Buffalo: Abundance, face problems head on, good luck

Wolf: Teacher medicine, determination, communication

Otter: Powerful energy, creativity, manifestation, resourcefulness

The West Direction is where the sun brings a balance to our days. The sun goes down to allow us to sleep and nourish our minds and bodies.

Spider: Limitless possibilities, psychic intuition, career choices

Turtle: Patience, endurance in difficult times, determination

Snake: New life, releasing the old, power to change

Man-in-the-Maze: Spiritual, emotional, physical balance, guidance

Kokopelli: Inspiration, creativity, fertility, sexuality

Eagle: Prayers answered, pride and courage, self-assessment

Bear: Strength, courage, overcome physical problems, self-reliance

Buffalo: Abundance, face problems head on, good luck

Wolf: Teacher medicine, determination, communication

Otter: Powerful energy, creativity, manifestation, resourcefulness

The North Direction is where the cold winds come from. They bring us relief from the hot summer and balance to the warmth.

Spider: Limitless possibilities, psychic intuition, career choices

Turtle: Patience, endurance in difficult times, determination

Snake: New life, releasing the old, power to change

Man-in-the-Maze: Spiritual, emotional, physical balance, guidance

Kokopelli: Inspiration, creativity, fertility, sexuality

Eagle: Prayers answered, pride and courage, self-assessment

Bear: Strength, courage, overcome physical problems, self-reliance

Buffalo: Abundance, face problems head on, good luck

Wolf: Teacher medicine, determination, communication

Otter: Powerful energy, creativity, manifestation, resourcefulness

The Above Direction is the home of the Creator and where the Eagle flies. From above comes our spiritual energy and above is where our prayers are answered.

Spider: Limitless possibilities, psychic intuition, career choices

Turtle: Patience, endurance in difficult times, determination

Snake: New life, releasing the old, power to change

Man-in-the-Maze: Spiritual, emotional, physical balance, guidance

Kokopelli: Inspiration, creativity, fertility, sexuality

Eagle: Prayers answered, pride and courage, self-assessment

Bear: Strength, courage, overcome physical problems, self-reliance

Buffalo: Abundance, face problems head on, good luck

Wolf: Teacher medicine, determination, communication

Otter: Powerful energy, creativity, manifestation, resourcefulness

The Below Direction is our Mother the Earth. It is the celestial body that is our home. The one that needs our love, respect, and protection; without her there is no life, for she gives us everything we need to live.

Spider: Limitless possibilities, psychic intuition, career choices

Turtle: Patience, endurance in difficult times, determination

Snake: New life, releasing the old, power to change

Man-in-the-Maze: Spiritual, emotional, physical balance, guidance

Kokopelli: Inspiration, creativity, fertility, sexuality

Eagle: Prayers answered, pride and courage, self-assessment

Bear: Strength, courage, overcome physical problems, self-reliance

Buffalo: Abundance, face problems head on, good luck

Wolf: Teacher medicine, determination, communication

Otter: Powerful energy, creativity, manifestation, resourcefulness

The Inner Direction is where our spiritual energy lives and learns. Our bodies should also have our love and respect, for it is a gift and a home for our spirits while they learn humbleness and to suffer.

Spider: Limitless possibilities, psychic intuition, career choices

Turtle: Patience, endurance in difficult times, determination

Snake: New life, releasing the old, power to change

Man-in-the-Maze: Spiritual, emotional, physical balance, guidance

Kokopelli: Inspiration, creativity, fertility, sexuality

Eagle: Prayers answered, pride and courage, self-assessment

Bear: Strength, courage, overcome physical problems, self-reliance

Buffalo: Abundance, face problems head on, good luck

Wolf: Teacher medicine, determination, communication

Otter: Powerful energy, creativity, manifestation, resourcefulness

SECTION IV

Summary of Stone People Medicine

From the technical side of stones and minerals, I know little. From the spiritual side I know much more, and I'm always learning. I've learned these simple practices pertaining to stones. Listen to them and you will receive answers to all your questions, and trust the answers the stones bring you. Once you see they do work, you will start to show respect. When you show respect, you begin to look at stones differently.

Soon this new way of treating stones carries over to the plants, animals, insects and other people. All the trees, plants, flowers and even weeds begin to receive your respect and you realize they also have a right to live and be here on this earth. They are such a big part of the balance.

We exhale carbon monoxide that gives them life and they pay us back by giving us the oxygen we need to survive. What a wonderful exchange! You may wonder what do plants have to do with stones. Even plants need stones.

Though we call it dirt, the smallest piece of earth no matter how microscopic, is still a stone. Stones always seem to arrange themselves in such a way to give the plants a strong base. When a tree has its roots into the earth, people believe it's the roots that are strong and are holding up the tree. Have you ever stopped to think that it is the arrangement of the stones that make it possible for the tree to remain standing? No matter how thick or long the roots are, if you remove the stones from around them the tree will fall.

The strength provided by the arrangement of the stones makes it possible for the plants to stay where they're growing during strong winds and storms. What the plants give the stones or the earth in return, is that their roots keep the stones from washing away and being rearranged. I believe when stones are moved by rain water or by any other natural means, it's because the stone has more knowledge to gather. Also by being rearranged, a stone that has to help someone would now be visible to that person.

When a person is compelled to pick up a stone, it is that stone's time to help and teach the individual drawn to it. Sometimes the person that picks it up is only being used by the stone so that it will be carried to the person that needs it. Have you ever been given a stone? That stone was looking for you. It used the person in a good way to bring and give it to you. It has a gift for you. Respect and treat it well. When you've received what you need from it, don't be surprised if you lose or suddenly decide to give it away.

As with other things we have a tendency to get attached to our little stone friends. Because you really like and even love a stone you can't believe your own actions as you contemplate giving it away. You might question yourself, asking why you are giving your favorite stone away. Its time to let the stone go to a new home. I believe the stone has given you what you need, now it has to help someone else. If you feel good about giving it away that means that you have certainly gained from having had the stone, whether you're aware of it or not.

If you are sad for having given it away, it's quite possible you weren't ready for the gift or knowledge that was being brought to you. Open yourself spiritually and rewards, gifts and knowledge shall be yours. With knowledge comes confidence, courage and limitless abilities. The confidence you gain is in yourself. Confidence to take long and more positive steps.

The courage comes from the confidence! You gain the courage to confront problems. Be they emotional, spiritual or otherwise. Courage to try to attain a better place in life. The limitless abilities are by products of your confidence and courage. Within this knowledge you stop putting limits on what you want to do. Then you feel you have gained one more valuable asset. Pride in yourself grows and grows every time something new enters your life. All this from just believing in a small stone that's come into your life!

This shouldn't seem complicated. It's so simple it's a wonder there's so many that need so much. They go through life, without the basic needs for a normal life. These people are the non-believers. They're the ones that think they know it all. They're the ones that scoff at the very idea that a stupid thing like a little stone can help them in any way! I feel sad for them. The way to use a stone to gain all you want is simple.

Read these next few sentences with a lot of care and believe. Hold whatever stone has come to you in the palm of your hand. If you want to talk out loud you may. If you want to convey your wishes and dreams to the stone through thoughts that's okay also. Hold it in your hands with respect, sincerity and simply talk to it as you will a good friend. Ask it the questions you want to be answered. For example you can ask it how you can make money. How you can change your personality, if you have a habit or some trait you don't like about yourself. Maybe you're overly bashful or you have a difficult time attracting nice people in your life for relationships. Anything you ask will be answered. Don't be impatient. Give the stone time to do its work. Give it time to help you unravel your problems. Stones in themselves are very powerful entities.

Spirit animals or guides are also very strong and helpful. The Great Spirit gave us both so we could use whichever a person preferred. You might ask which is the stronger of the two. The only way I know to answer that is by a few questions of my own.

Which one feels good to you, the spirit animal or the stone?

Which came to you first, a spirit animal or a stone?

Do you like a certain stone or do you feel an affinity to some animal?

These are very important questions you should answer in order for you to learn what will be best for you. It will show you where you can most gain from it.

I want to get into just a little about the difference between the two.

A rock is your common everyday rock you walk on type of earth. A stone is a piece of the same earth but we deem it to have some kind of value. So doesn't it mean in fact that a common little rock can become a stone to you? Does a value always have to be fronted by a dollar sign? I believe like beauty, value is only in the eye or feeling of the person holding the little stone or rock.

The dictionary describes rock as -- a large mass of stone -- broken pieces of stone.

The dictionary describes stone as -- the hard, solid, nonmetallic mineral matter of rock -- a piece of rock.

Meaning any stone or rock coming to you, possesses the power to help you. They are one and the same.

Does the size of stone or rock have any added value? In my opinion, not more monetary value, but perhaps if it's bigger it might contain more information than a small one. But for a second remember what I've said before. You'll be attracted to a stone if it has something for you.

Sometimes you could be at a special place outdoors. Maybe at a picnic area or perhaps in a place you're getting to know someone better. Maybe you're on vacation somewhere and want to capture the moment. You can pick up a small stone, and take it with you. The stone will forever hold that moment or time that was special to you. And when times are difficult you can take that stone out and let it take you back to a better, happier time. This is another way stones can be there for you. Some people carry a bag of special stones with them, each one contains a special moment or memory from the past.

I've never said anything about size or appearance, because it's not relevant. The stone that has information for you might not be one you can pick up and carry with you. It might be a stone you go to, to ask questions when your need arises. You might find a Stone people friend that is located in your favorite spot where you like to sit and meditate or just contemplate. It might be a favorite spot in your back yard. Did you ever stop to think it might be a stone there making it such a pleasant place?

Have you ever talked to people who love to climb cliffs? There are those who become obsessed with climbing a sheer wall of rock, picking the hardest ones to attempt climbing. Why is this? It's more than an obsession. It almost becomes a spiritual conquest or endeavor. They almost worship the rock, the challenge. Just for a minute, ask yourself why? Why do they do this? Why do they place themselves in danger of falling and getting killed or hurt? Maybe they are drawn to do this because the rock has a lesson to teach them. Perhaps the lesson is one of courage. Maybe they must learn about their own strengths and weaknesses.

Those high precipices have always been honored by the native people. The huge single pieces of rock are so enormous they possess special places for spiritual guidance. They are also always close to the Great Spirit, therefore high rocky places make excellent spots to "cry for visions and guidance," to vision quest.

Can you imagine the amount of knowledge that could be yours from places as grand as that? A person could live by such a place and make it into a place of worship like the old people did. At the same time volumes could be filled with the knowledge gained from the giant stone. It is willing to give up what it knows to a true believer and a good listener.

I don't mean every rock you see laying on the ground has a significant meaning for you. This does not mean you can't pick up a rock to scare off some mean dog trying to bite you. That you can't pick up a small flat stone and try to see how many times you can skip it across the lake. I don't mean that you should load yourself down with so many rocks and stones, they become a burden to you. Most rocks and stones in the world were created, simply to hold the world in place. Not every stone you see has a message for you. Those you have a strong compulsion to pick up or are strongly drawn to, are the ones you should be concerned with.

The rocks and stones we walk on have been given a job by the creator. The job of giving us a strong world or base to walk on.

For native people the stones have forever been significant and have been our relatives. They have helped us survive by making life easier. We have used them as tools, decorations, weapons and as a means of communication. They were our books and our libraries. We used the stones in caves to tell our brothers that came after us what we were doing. Whether we had plenty to eat or not. Only people with full stomachs take the time to express their feelings through art, and take time to tell their stories of success. So every time we see petroglyphs on cave walls or on stones, we know the old people that lived there were happy, well fed and content.

As an elder and from what I've done in my life spiritually, I have earned the right and privilege to counsel others. My thoughts, advice and counsel are within these pages and are meant only to help others.

As mentioned the "Stone Man" is

picked by the spirits through dreams. Their job is to supply stones to people that need them. I have accepted that responsibility because I too, am a "Stone Man".

We should be deeply grateful to the creator, who gave us life to share with this piece of the universe. The creator has seen fit to place humans on an equal basis to stone. He has given all of us the same right to live.

Hopefully what you have learned within these pages will serve as a guide to raise your spirituality and your place in life. My deepest wish is you appreciate and let stones into your life to serve you as they were meant to.

Should you find that your favorite store carries this book, but not our other products,

Wo-Pila Publishing has other items to offer.

If you wish to order any of the Stone People Medicine stones write to the address below. They are $5.00 each, plus .50 shipping per stone. Check or money orders should be payable to Wo-Pila Publishing.

We also carry other handmade native crafts including:
Stop Smoking the Native Way tape
Medicine Wheels, Dream Catchers, Crystal necklaces & earrings, Drums, Rattles, Medicine bags, Prayer sticks, etc. Write or call for a catalog of these items.

Wo-Pila Publishing
P.O. Box 84002
Phoenix, Az. 85071-4002

1-800-STONE-22